Q & A

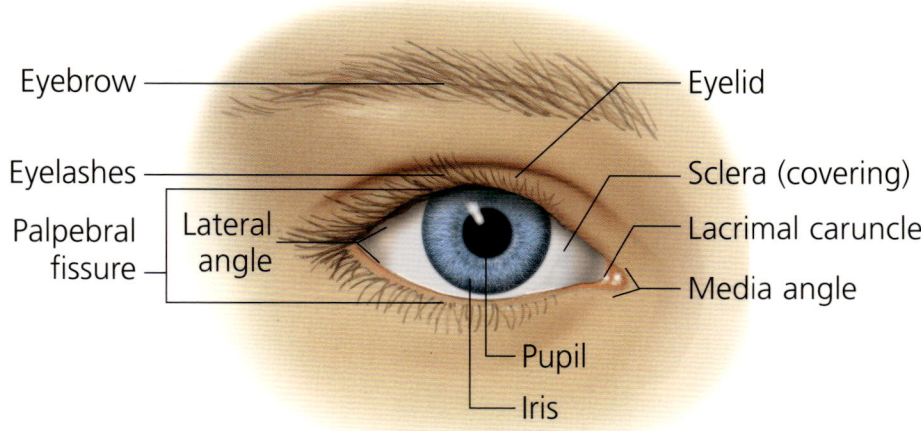

What is the eye?

The eye is one of the most important of our sensory organs. Often referred to as "the windows to the soul," the eyes are the organs which allow us **stereoscopic vision** (depth perception), an adaptation to the environment which ensured our survival. Our eyes receive a stimulus from light reflected off an object, and **photoreceptors** in the eye convert this light energy into nerve impulses. Only the visible light portion of the electromagnetic spectrum can trigger these photoreceptors. The brain interprets these signals and gives an accurate analysis of form, light intensity, color, and movement.

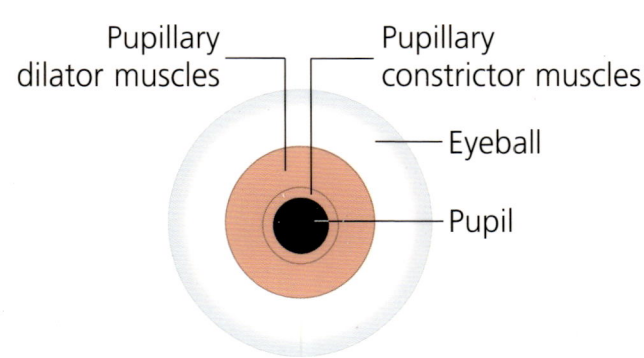

Pupillary muscle action

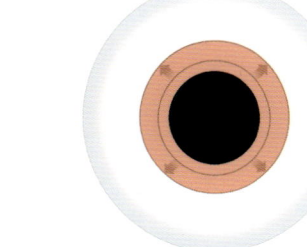

Bright light — Constrictor contracts, narrowing the pupil

Low light — Dilator contracts, widening the pupil

The accessory structures of the eye

The **eyelids** protect the eye from injury and prevent it from drying out. They distribute the fluid, called tears, that is secreted and drained by the **lacrimal apparatus**. The **eyebrows** and **eyelashes** both protect the eye from airborne and falling particles. The **conjunctiva**, a mucous membrane lining the inside of the eyelids and continuing around the front of the eyeball, prevents objects from sliding around to the back of the eye.

Each eye sits in a bony depression of the skull, the **orbit**, which protects and supports the eye while providing a place for attachment for the **extrinsic ocular muscles**, the six muscles that control the movement of the eye.

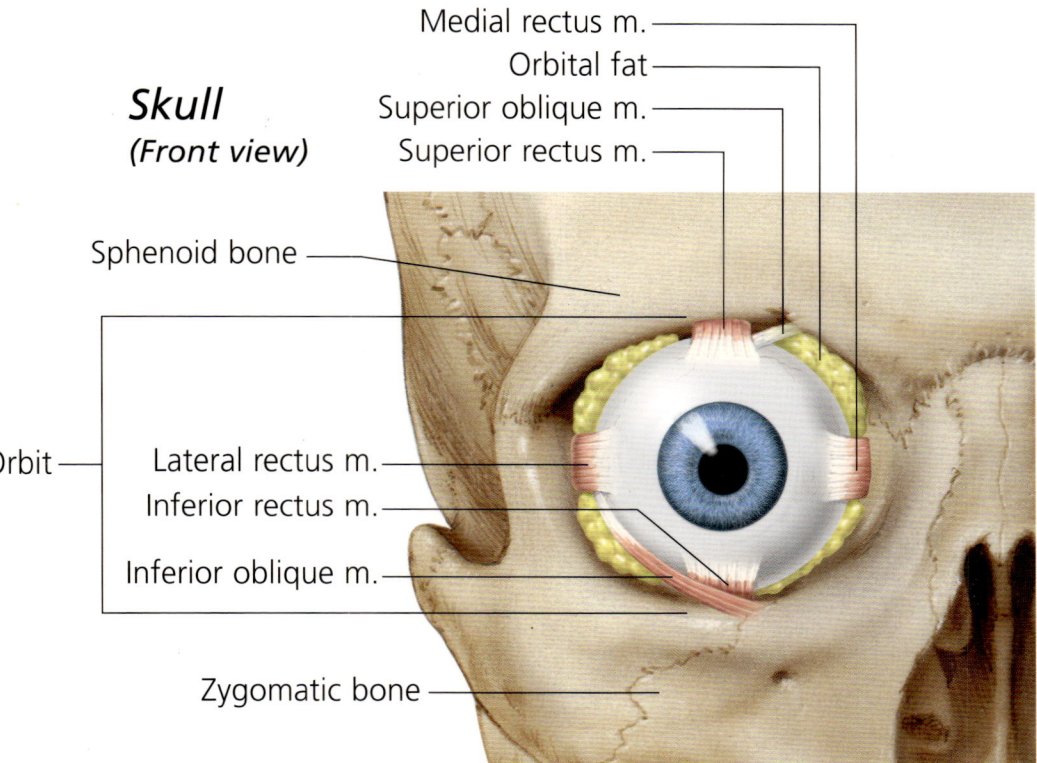

Skull (Front view)

Key of abbreviations
m. Muscle

The iris and pupil

The opening in the iris is called the **pupil**. In the iris two different smooth muscles control the size of the pupil, which determines the amount of light reaching the lens. Constriction is under parasympathetic fiber control, while dilation is controlled by sympathetic fibers. A protective reaction that constricts the pupils, called the **pupillary light reflex**, occurs when a bright light suddenly hits the eyes.

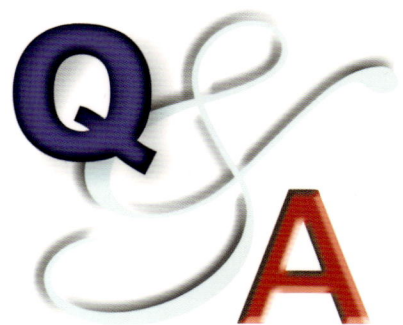

What is the scleral venous sinus?

The **aqueous humor** produced by the ciliary body provides nutrients for the lens and cornea, and helps maintain the pressure in the front of the eye. Aqueous humor is reabsorbed back into the bloodstream through the **scleral venous sinus** (Canal of Schlemm), located at the junction of the sclera and cornea.

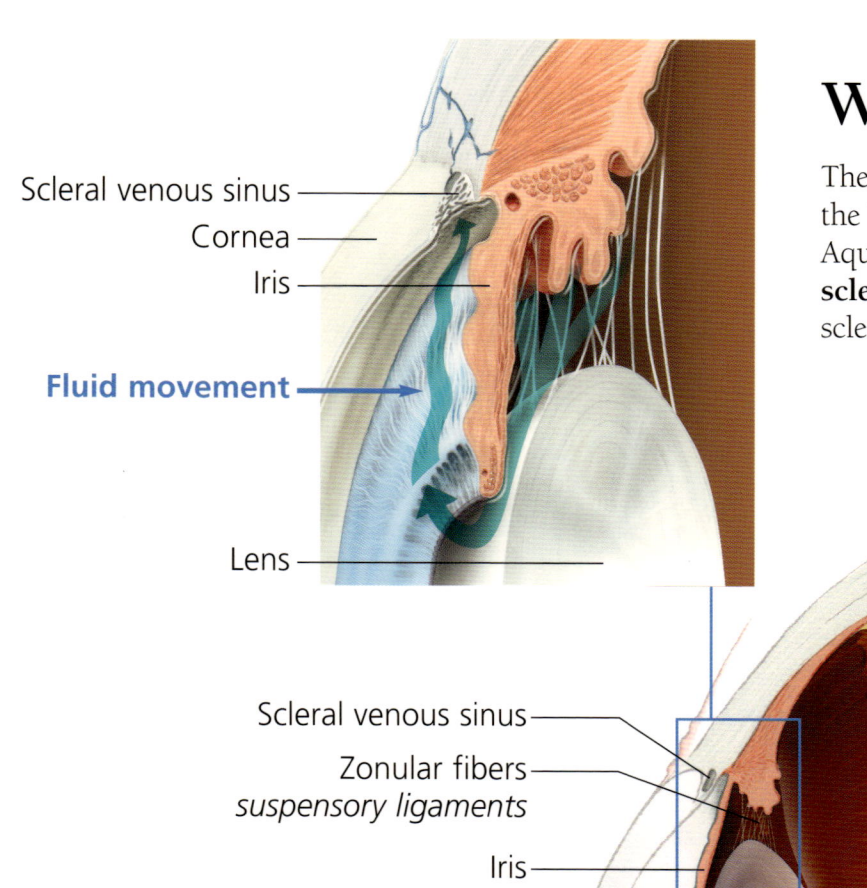

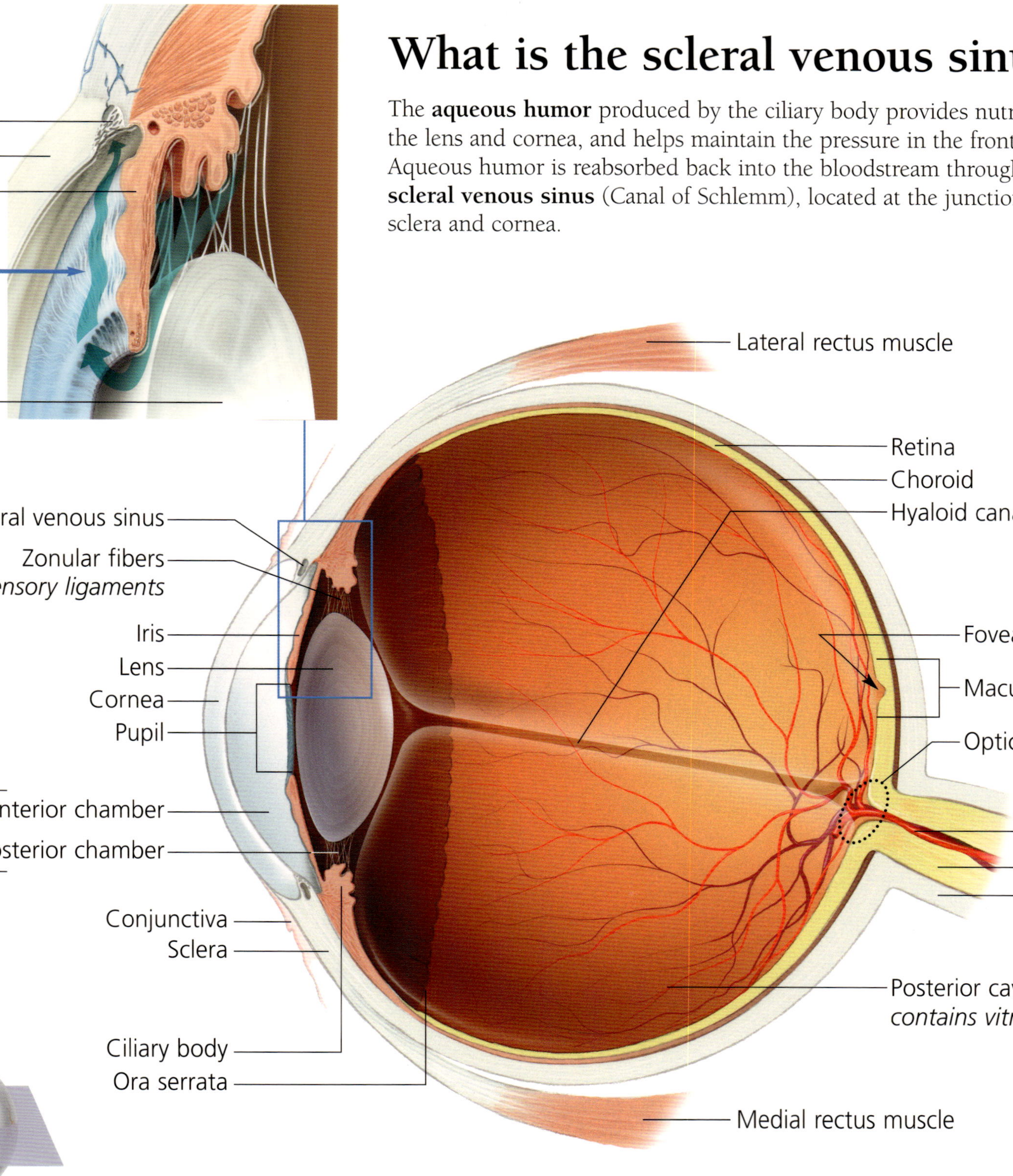

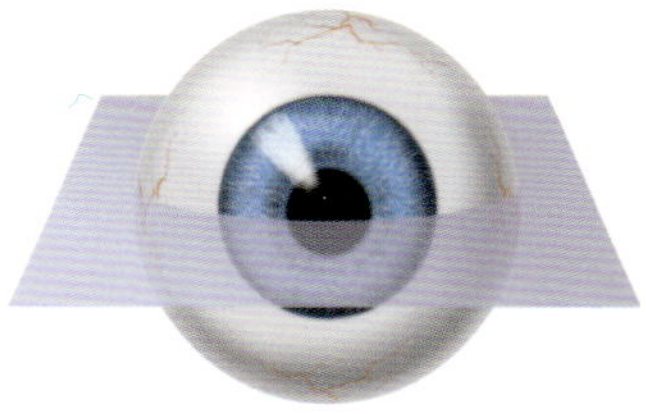

Right eye (Transverse section)

The structures of the eyeball

The wall of the eyeball is made up of three layers. The outermost layer, the **fibrous tunic**, contains both the **sclera** (gives shape to the eyeball) and the **cornea** (transmits and refracts light). The middle layer, the **vascular tunic**, is made up of the **choroid** (supplies blood to the eye), the **ciliary body** (supports the **lens** and produces a fluid called the **aqueous humor**) and the **iris** (regulates the amount of light by controlling **pupil** size). The innermost layer, the **internal tunic**, contains the **retina** (provides photoreception and transmits impulses). Within the eyeball and suspended from the ciliary body by the **suspensory ligament** is the **lens**, which refracts and focuses the light onto the retina.

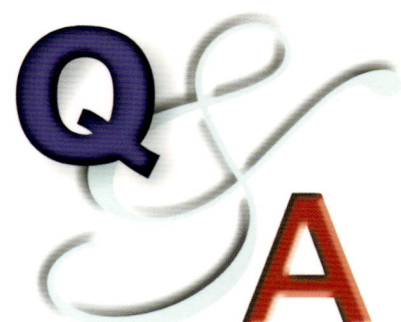

What is the retina?

The **retina**, the internal tunic, is in the posterior part of the eyeball. It is made up of two layers, the **pigmented layer** and the **nervous layer**. The nervous layer is made of three layers of neurons: ganglion cells, bipolar neurons, and photoreceptors. When light hits the retina, it strikes the ganglion cell layer first and then passes through the bipolar layer before reaching the photoreceptors, the **rods** and **cones**. The 120 million rods are the most sensitive to light while the 6 million cones provide color vision and greater visual acuity.

Fovea centralis

The **fovea centralis** is a small pit within the yellow area of the retina called the **macula lutea**. Visual acuity is greatest in the fovea because the area contains only cones and, due to the structure, is the only spot of the retina where light directly hits these photoreceptors.

Optic disc

The **optic disc** is where the nerve fibers from the retina gather together to exit the eye as the **optic nerve**. The disc lacks photoreceptors and is called the eye's blind spot.

Retina
(membrane lining the back of the eye)

- A. Fovea centralis
- a. Macula lutea
- B. Superior nasal artery
- C. Inferior nasal artery
- D. Superior nasal artery
- E. Inferior nasal artery
- F. Central retinal artery
- G. Optic nerve

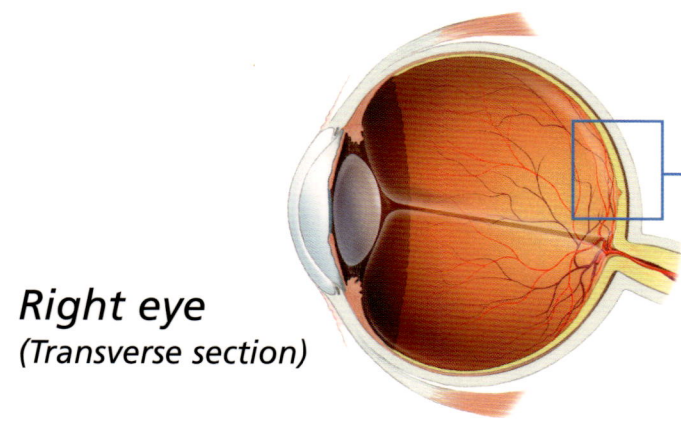

Right eye
(Transverse section)

Rods and cones

What are rods and cones?

The two kinds of photoreceptors, **rods** and **cones**, so called because of their shapes, are specialized neurons (nerve cells). They generate a nerve impulse when stimulated by light. Rods and cones connect to bipolar cells, which then connect ganglion cells. The axons of the ganglion cells come together to form the optic nerve. One group of ganglion cells, directly connecting to the brain, detects changes in light during a day/night cycle, helping to establish our circadian rhythms.

Rods are more numerous, about 120 million, compared to cones, numbering about 6 million. Rods are very sensitive to light and can function in dim light. They provide black and white imaging while cones provide sharp color vision. Cone cells come in three kinds, each carrying a different pigment. Each kind is sensitive to one region of the visible light spectrum (red, green, or blue).

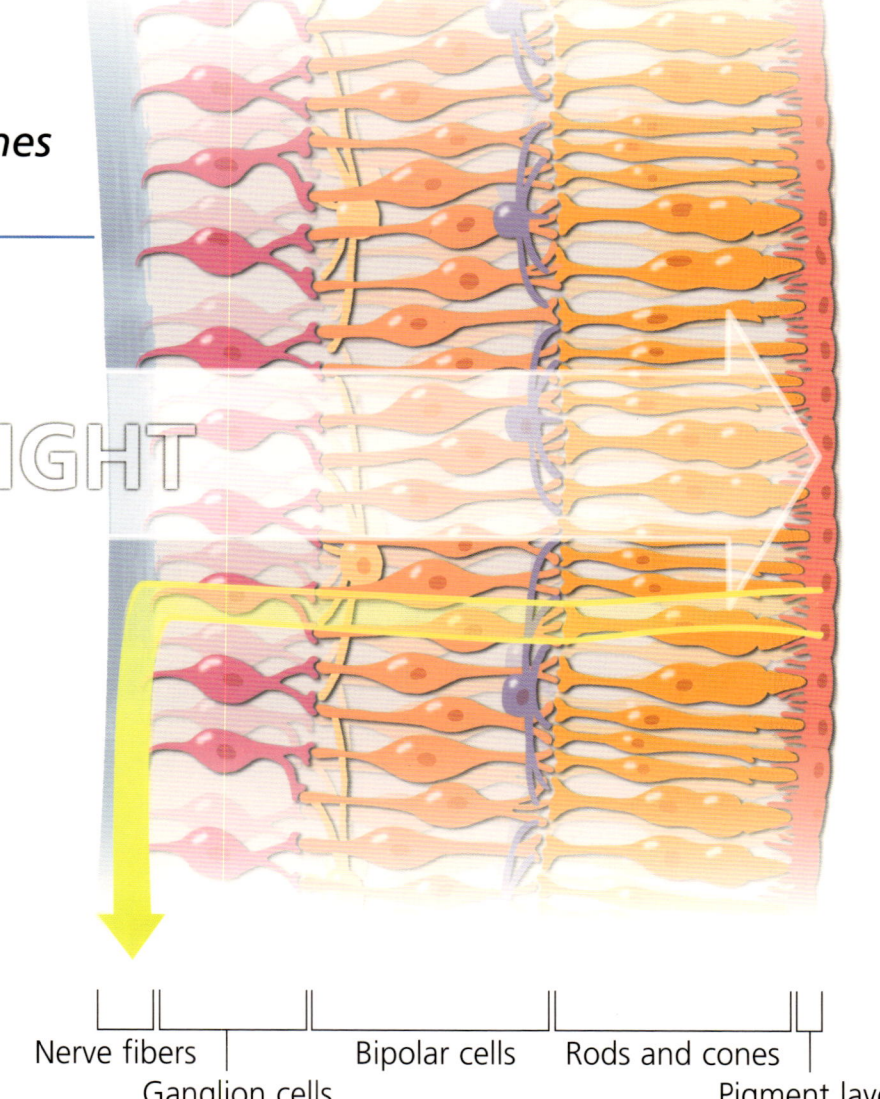

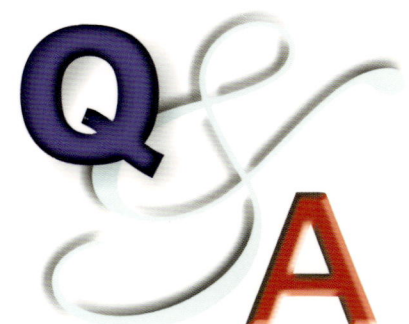

What is light?

Most life on our planet depends on light. The **electromagnetic spectrum**, a huge, continuous range of radiation, includes the familiar range of visible light. Radiation travels in waves, measured in **wavelengths**. Red light, at one end of the visible light range, has a longer wavelength than purple, at the other end. Infrared radiation has a longer wavelength than red light, so we don't see it, but we feel it as heat. At the other end of the visible light range is purple light, with a shorter wavelength than red. Ultraviolet radiation has an even shorter wavelength, so we don't see it.

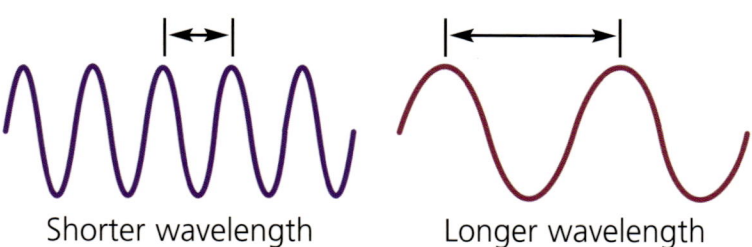

Shorter wavelength   Longer wavelength

Key to wavelength
Nanometer = One billionth of a meter

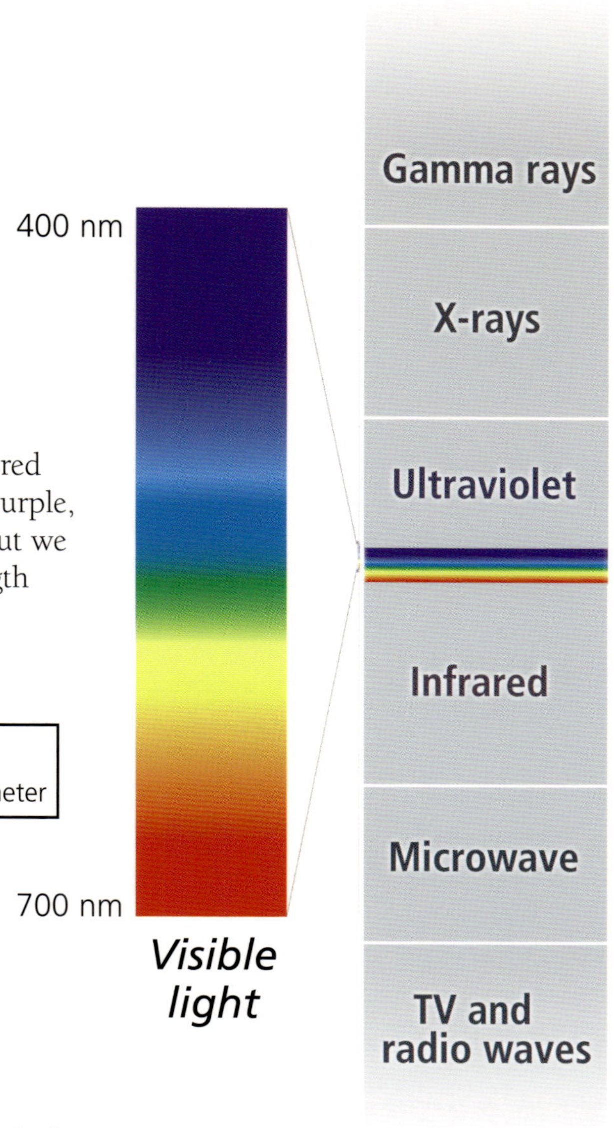

400 nm

700 nm

Visible light

Gamma rays

X-rays

Ultraviolet

Infrared

Microwave

TV and radio waves

Electromagnetic spectrum

What is vision?

The eyes receive a stimulus from light reflected from an object and photoreceptors in the eye convert this light energy into nerve impulses. Only part of the spectrum of light, called **visible light**, can trigger these photoreceptors—wavelengths between 400 and 700 nanometers. The brain interprets these signals and gives an accurate analysis of form, light intensity, color, and movement.

What is ultraviolet (UV) radiation?

Light waves from 400 nm to 90 nm (nanometers) are classified as **ultraviolet (UV) radiation** and are invisible to the human eye. Sunlight is the primary source of UV radiation to which humans are exposed. The eye filters some UV radiation, but long exposures can cause vision problems.

Over-exposure to UVA and UVB radiation can have a negative and often irreversible impact on your eye health. UVC radiation is absorbed by the ozone layer and does not impact us.

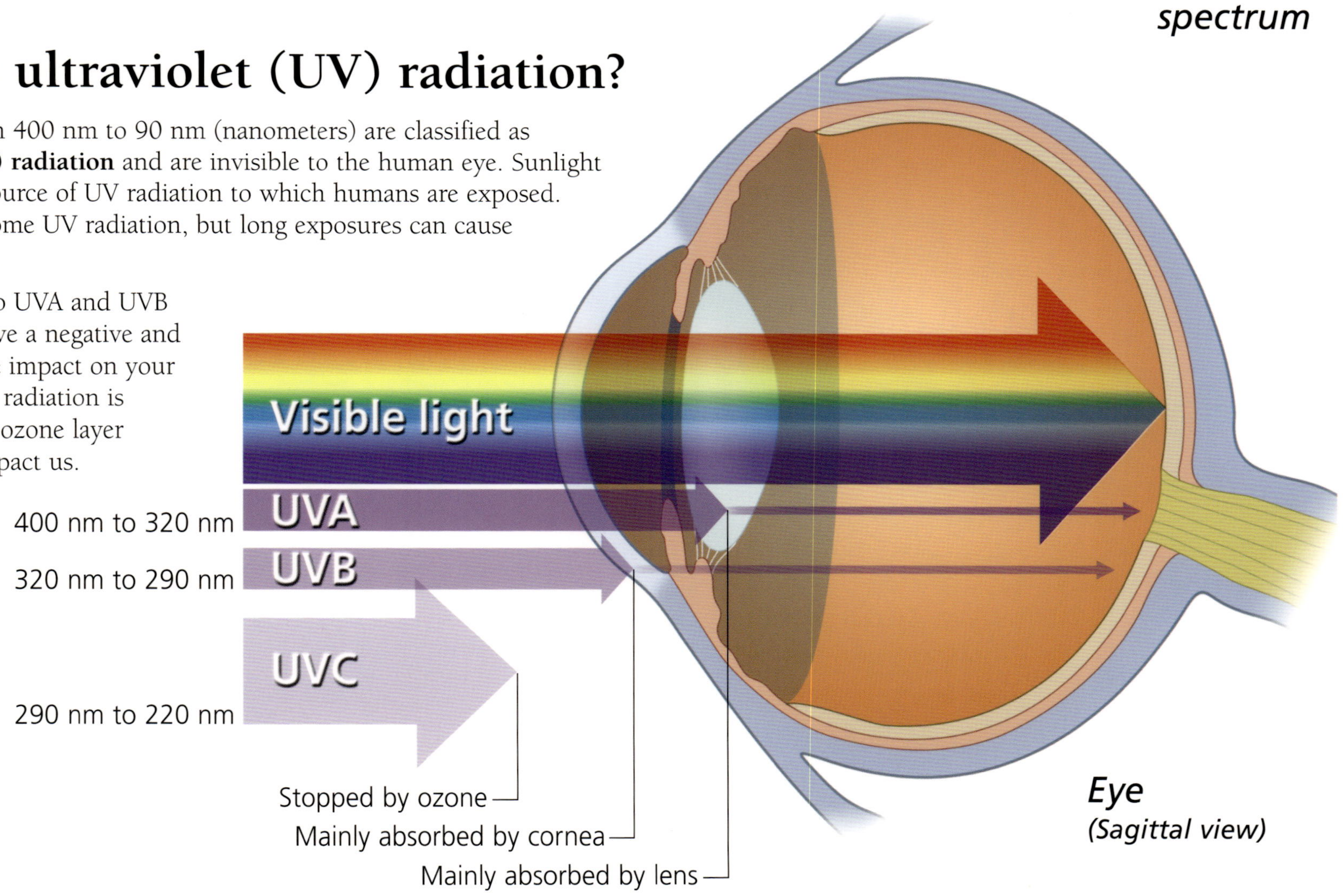

Visible light

400 nm to 320 nm UVA
320 nm to 290 nm UVB
290 nm to 220 nm UVC

Stopped by ozone
Mainly absorbed by cornea
Mainly absorbed by lens

Eye (Sagittal view)

Understanding the Eye

Q & A

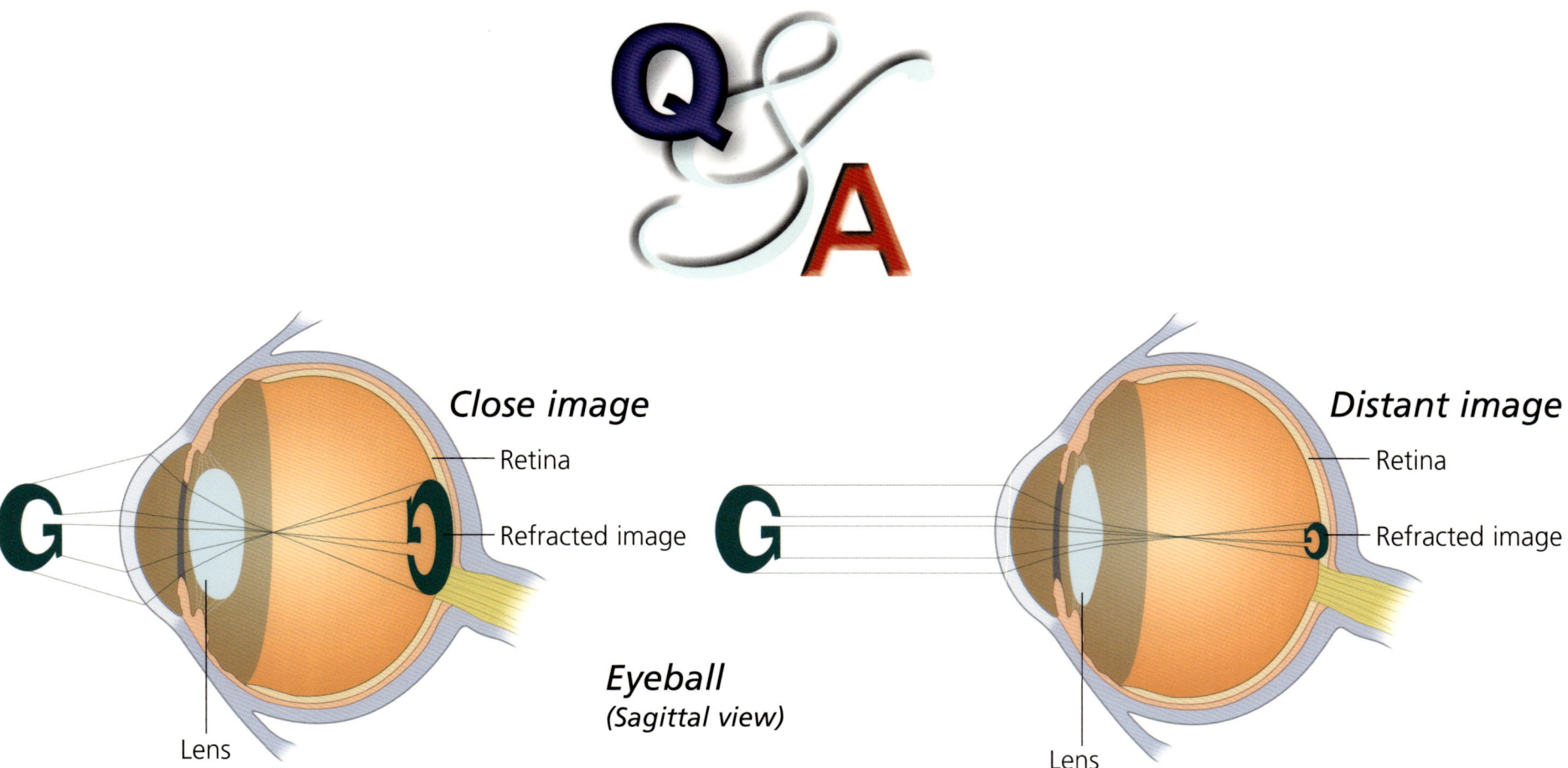

What is accommodation?

The ability of the eye to keep an image focusing on the retina is called **accommodation**. When light enters the eye, light is **refracted**, or bent, to focus onto the retina. In order to keep nearby objects in focus, the eye has to adjust this refraction. It does this by changing the shape of the lens by use of the **ciliary zonule**. This muscular ring either contracts, making the lens less round, or relaxes, making the lens more rounded.

Refraction issues

Light is focused through the cornea and lens, forming an image on the retina. If this process (accommodation) malfunctions, our vision is disrupted.

Myopia, or nearsightedness, happens when the eyeballs are longer than normal. The image is focused in front of the retina, producing a fuzzy image. A concave (diverging) corrective lens moves the focal point backward so the image is focused on the retina.

Hyperopia, or farsightedness, happens when the eyeballs are shorter than normal. The image is focused behind the retina, producing a fuzzy image. A convex (converging) corrective lens moves the focal point forward so the image is focused on the retina.

Astigmatism occurs when there are irregular or unequal curvatures with the lens or cornea. The light rays are not focused in one place, producing a fuzzy or distorted image. This condition can be corrected with contact lenses or glasses.

Key to illustrations
- - - - - Shape of normal eye

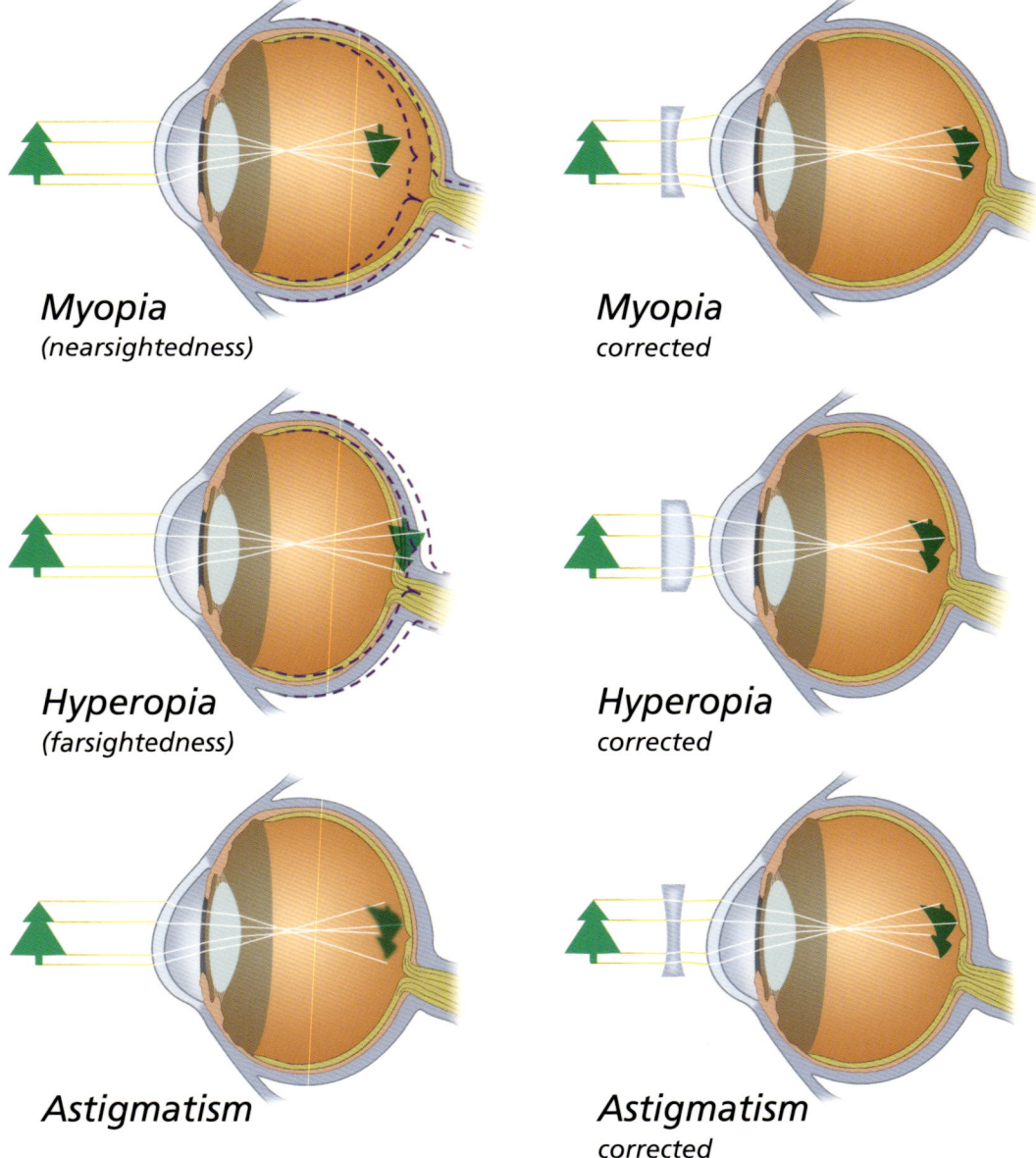

Q & A

Visual pathways

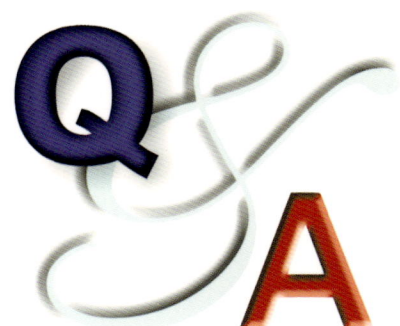

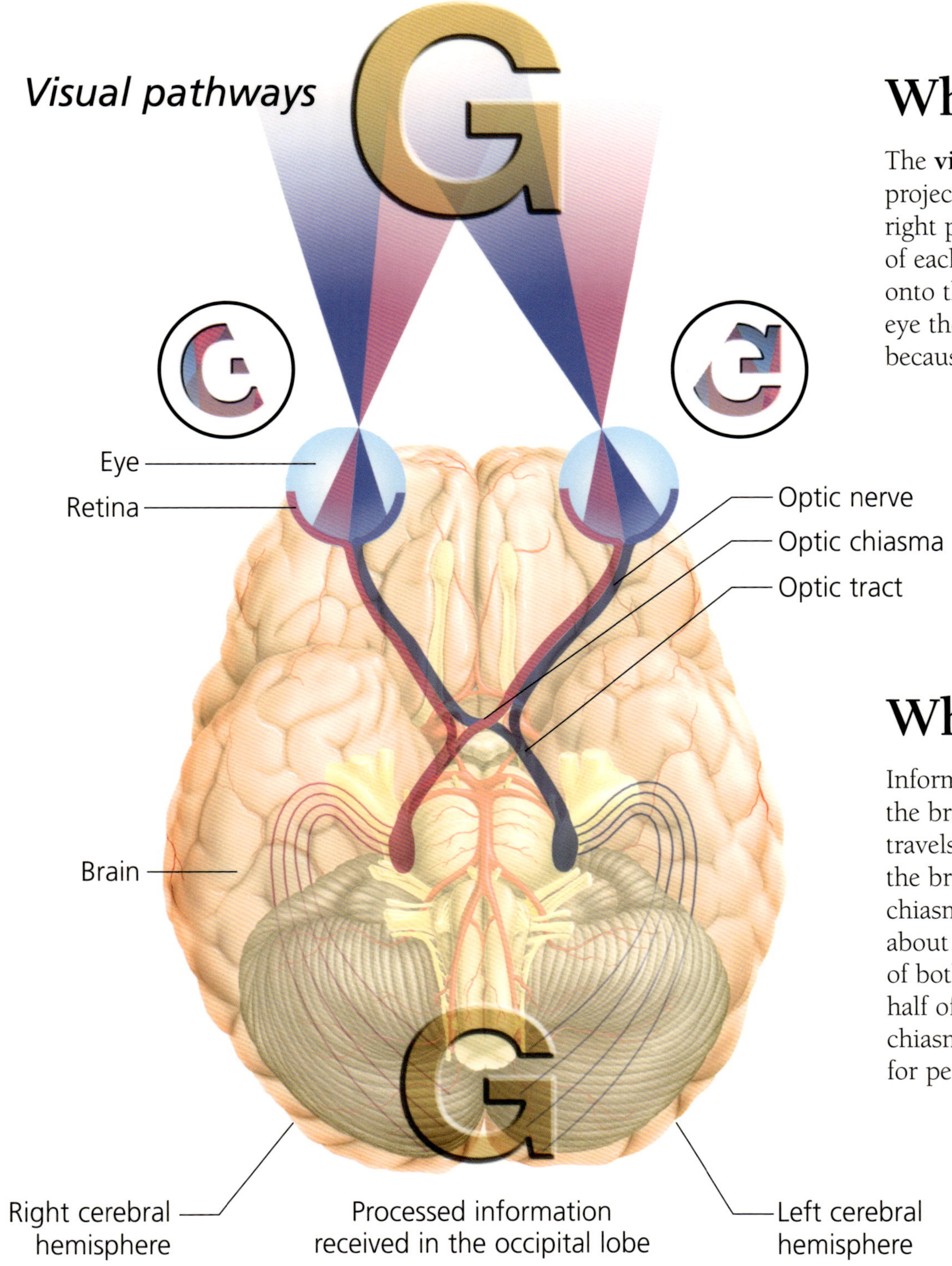

- Eye
- Retina
- Optic nerve
- Optic chiasma
- Optic tract
- Brain
- Right cerebral hemisphere
- Processed information received in the occipital lobe
- Left cerebral hemisphere

What is a visual field?

The **visual field** is the part of the external world that is projected onto the retina. The cornea and lens focus the right part of the visual field onto the left part of the retina of each eye, and the left part of the visual field is focused onto the right part of the retina of each eye. Within each eye the visual field is projected upside down and reversed because of refraction.

What are visual pathways?

Information about the visual field travels from the retinas to the brain. Information from the right side of the visual field travels from the left halves of both retinas to the left side of the brain. Half of the signals from the left eye cross the optic chiasma to reach the right side of the brain. Information about the left side of the visual field hits the right halves of both retinas and travels to the right side of the brain — half of the signals from the right eye also cross at the optic chiasma. Within the brain, signals travel to areas responsible for perception and eye and body movements.

Functional areas of the brain

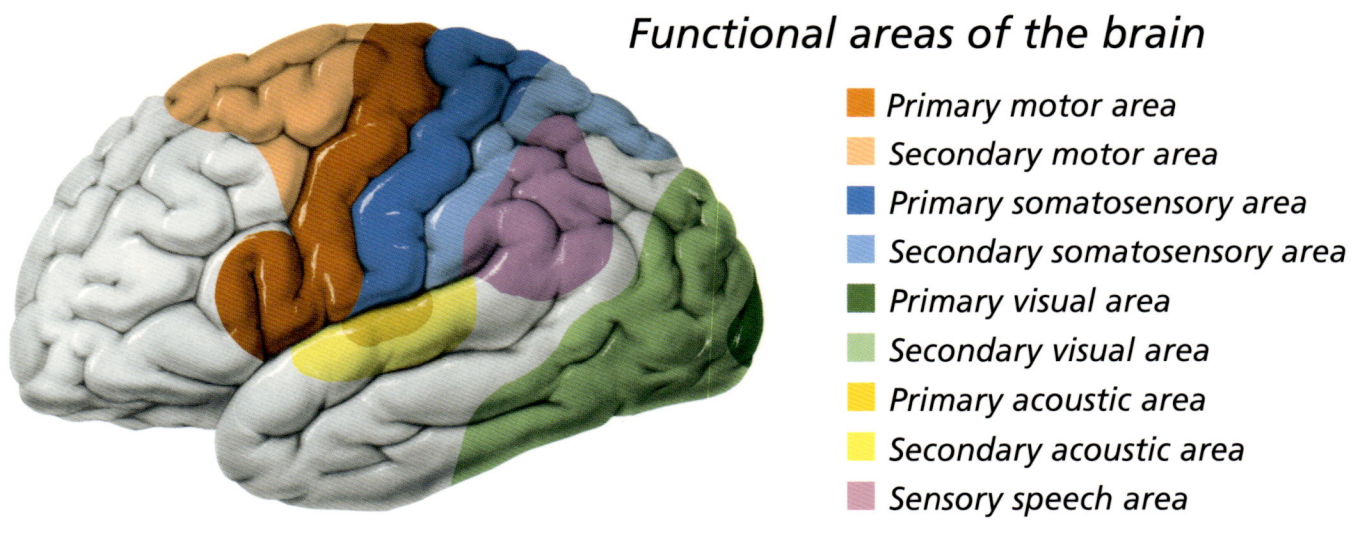

- Primary motor area
- Secondary motor area
- Primary somatosensory area
- Secondary somatosensory area
- Primary visual area
- Secondary visual area
- Primary acoustic area
- Secondary acoustic area
- Sensory speech area

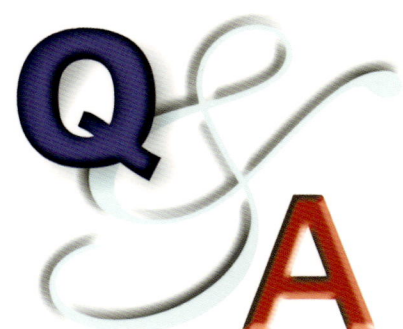

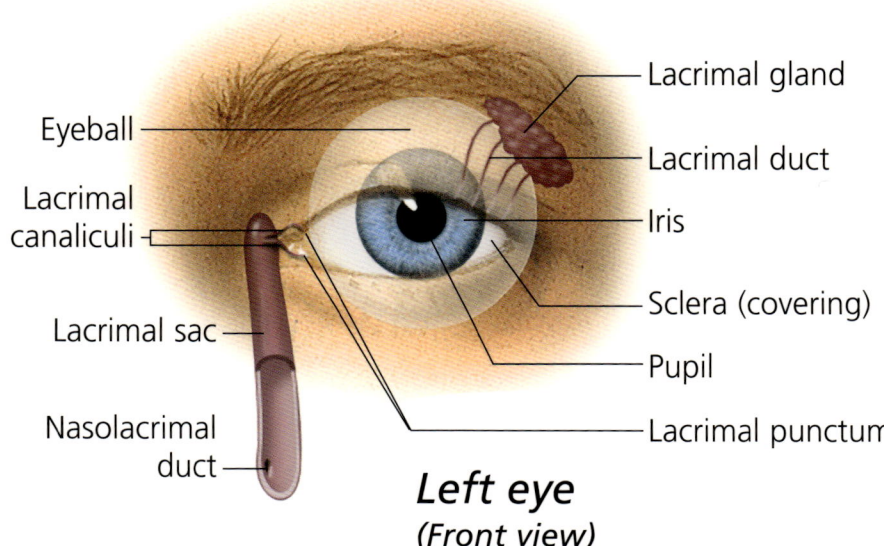

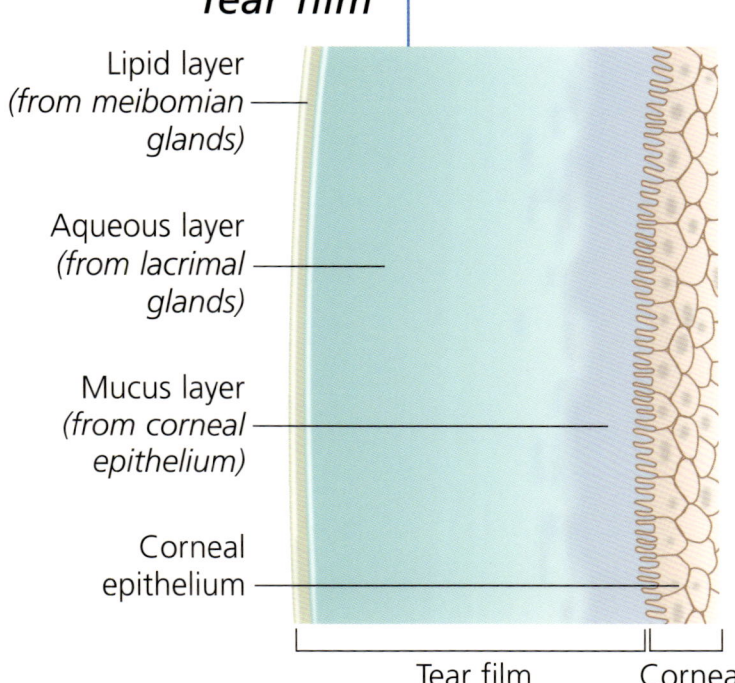

What is dry eye?

Dry eye is a disorder involving tears and the surface of the eye. Normally the constant flow of tears washes away particles and debris, helps prevent bacterial infections, and reduces friction by lubricating the eye. In dry eye multiple causes can contribute to an insufficiency of tears needed to moisten and protect the eye surface.

Dry eye syndrome (keratoconjunctivitis sicca) occurs when there is a deficiency in any of the layers of the tear film. DES involves the interaction of several factors: inadequate production of tears, increased evaporation of tears, and changes in the make-up of the tear film.

Symptoms of dry eye can include reduction in visual acuity; sensations of burning, stinging, or grittiness; ocular fatigue, even after short periods of reading; and **photophobia** (extreme sensitivity to light).

Causes of dry eye

While anyone can develop dry eye, the condition frequently affects the elderly. Dry eye is more prevalent in women than men, particularly post menopausal women. Dry eye can result from a single factor or a combination of reasons.

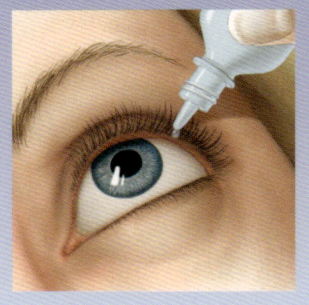

How is dry eye diagnosed?

Determining the cause of dry eye involves a comprehensive eye examination. The patient's history will help evaluate possible causes of dry eye, including medical conditions, current medications, and environmental factors. Testing would focus on tear production, the quantity and quality of tears, the tear layer, and the determination of the type of dry eye.

How is dry eye treated?

Treatment of dry eye depends on the underlying cause or causes. Treatments can involve the addition of artificial tears, procedures to help conserve tears, and medication and nutritional supplements to aid in the production of tears. Treatment options include:
- Topical application of artificial tears (tear substitutes)
- Environmental changes:
  – adjusting the air flow at home, the office and in vehicles
  – adjusting the humidity to control dryness
  – avoiding pollutants such as cigarette smoke, including second-hand smoke
- Correcting physical problems, such as eyelids not closing properly
- Including nutritional elements in the diet (Omega-3, fish and flaxseed oils)
- Surgical procedures, such as punctal occlusion and tarsorrhaphy

Q & A

What is glaucoma?

Glaucoma is a group of diseases marked by progressive damage to the optic nerve. An increase in the pressure of the fluid inside the eyes (**intraocular pressure**, or IOP) is a common feature. This increase can lead to loss of vision, and possibly to blindness if the condition is left untreated. It is more common and may be more severe in African-Americans and in people with a family history of the disease. The most common form of the disease is open angle glaucoma, which affects about two-thirds of glaucoma sufferers. Less common is closed-angle glaucoma, a serious condition that can occur suddenly or develop over a period of time. One type of open-angle glaucoma is characterized by a normal IOP.

Fluid movement

Fluid normally passes through a narrow space between the iris and lens, then drains out of the eye through the trabecular meshwork. The fluid continues draining through the scleral venous sinus before returning to the venous system. If this outward flow is blocked, or there is too much fluid, the resulting increase in pressure can damage the optic nerve and reduce vision.

The eye
(Sagittal section)

- Scleral venous sinus
- Inadequate aqueous drainage
- Iris
- Aqueous drainage through the pupil

Open-angle glaucoma
Closed-angle glaucoma

- Pupillary blockage
- Iris
- Aqueous drainage is blocked by the iris
- Scleral venous sinus

Detail of normal retina

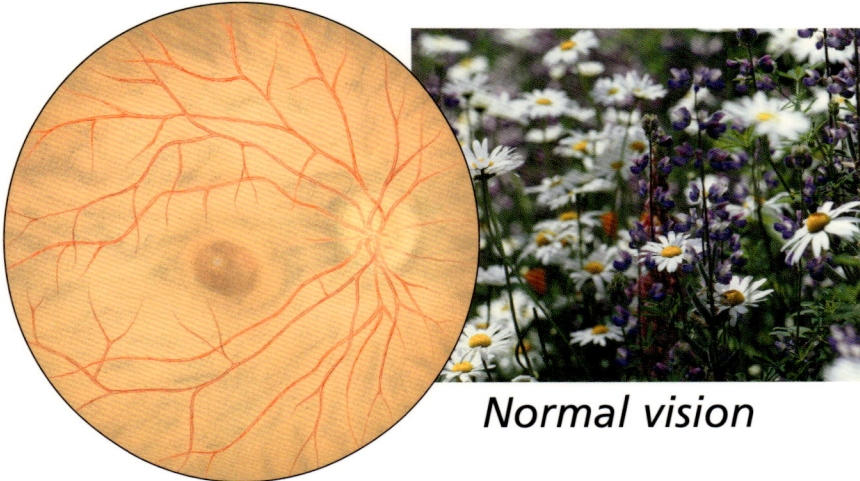

Normal vision

Detail of retina with glaucoma

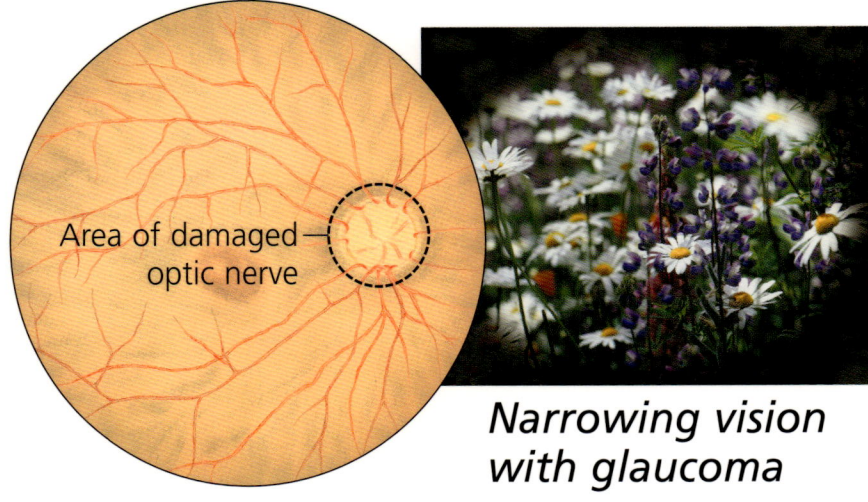

Area of damaged optic nerve

Narrowing vision with glaucoma

Risk factors for glaucoma

Glaucoma affects more than two million Americans and more than 70 million people worldwide. Risk factors include:

- Age (Risk of developing glaucoma increases after the age of 50)
- Race (African-Americans are three to four times more likely to develop glaucoma)
- Family history of glaucoma
- Medical conditions (i.e., diabetes, high blood pressure, or heart disease)
- Certain medications (i.e., corticosteroids, antihypertensives, and antihistamines)
- Trauma and injury to the eye

At first, people with glaucoma are free of symptoms. Vision is normal, and there is no pain associated with the condition. As the disease progresses, people may have difficulty moving from a bright room into a darker one and in judging steps and curbs. A person with glaucoma may continue to see objects directly in front of him clearly. However, objects to the side (periphery) may be missed. Blindness can result from a progressive loss of visual field if the disease remains untreated.

Q & A

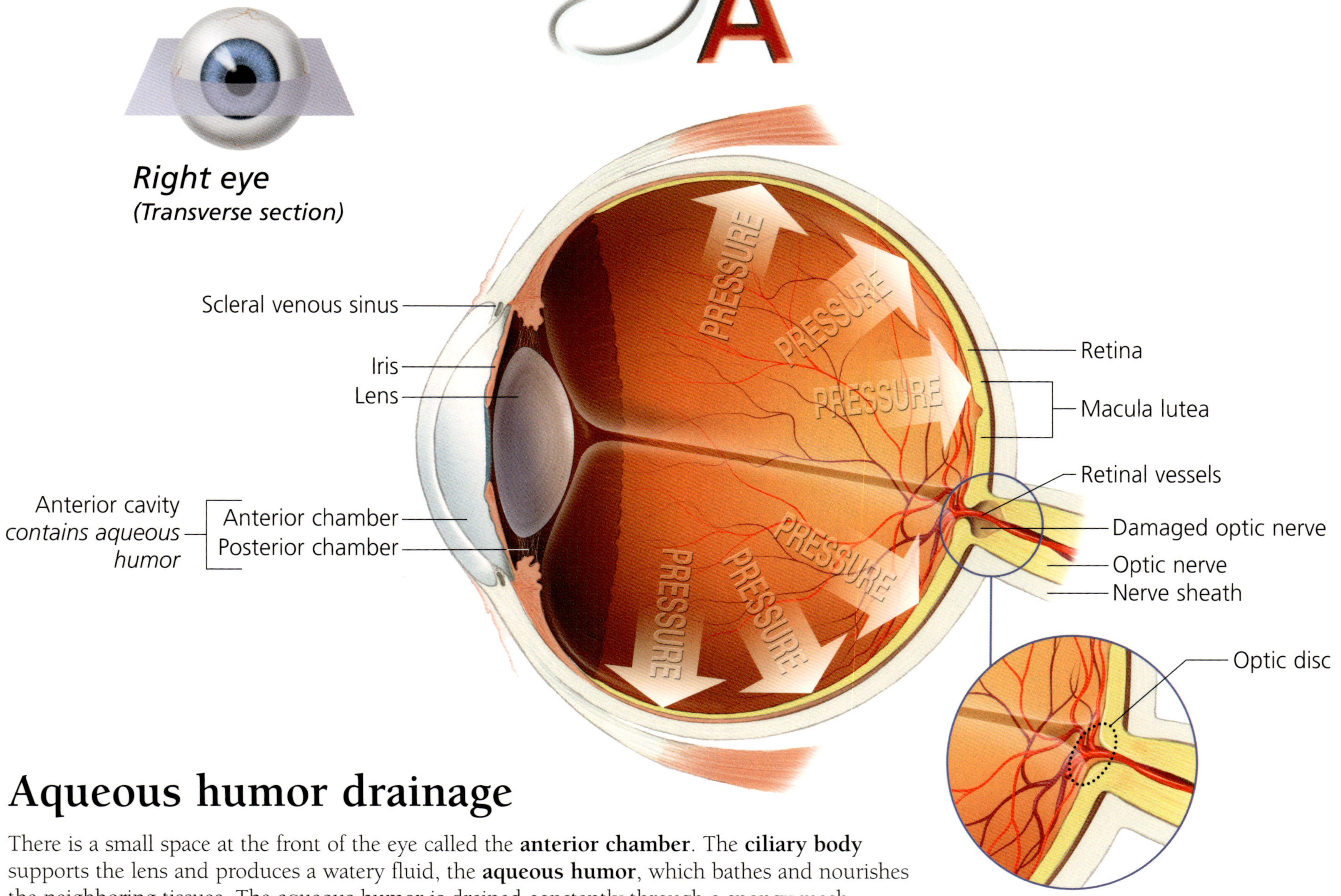

Right eye
(Transverse section)

- Scleral venous sinus
- Iris
- Lens
- Anterior cavity *contains aqueous humor*
  - Anterior chamber
  - Posterior chamber
- Retina
- Macula lutea
- Retinal vessels
- Damaged optic nerve
- Optic nerve
- Nerve sheath
- Optic disc

Cross section of normal optic nerve

Aqueous humor drainage

There is a small space at the front of the eye called the **anterior chamber**. The **ciliary body** supports the lens and produces a watery fluid, the **aqueous humor**, which bathes and nourishes the neighboring tissues. The aqueous humor is drained constantly through a spongy mesh (trabecular meshwork) that lies in the angle between the iris and the inner surface of the cornea, then into the scleral venous sinus. If the meshwork is blocked, or there is an overproduction of fluid, the fluid can drain too slowly, causing the intraocular pressure to increase. These changes can cause damage to the retina, resulting in defects in vision.

How is glaucoma diagnosed and treated?

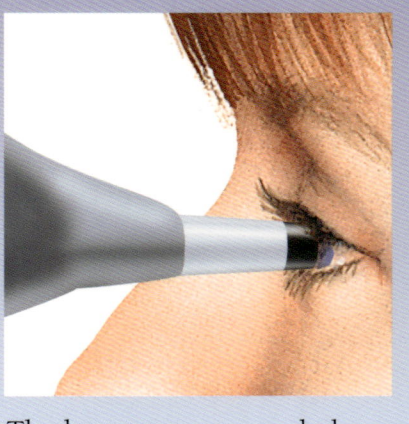

Glaucoma is a chronic disease that develops slowly. Damage to the optic nerve and visual loss can develop in many patients before the condition has been diagnosed. Regular eye examinations are essential for people who are at risk of developing glaucoma and for those who have been diagnosed with the disease.

High intraocular pressure (IOP) increases a person's risk of developing glaucoma, but does not mean that the person has the disease. The development of glaucoma in an individual depends upon the level of intraocular pressure that the optic nerve will tolerate. Some people with glaucoma have a normal IOP.

A range of tests can be used to diagnose and monitor glaucoma. Factors in diagnosis include IOP measurement, examination of the optic nerve, and vision field defects.

The best way to control glaucoma is to ensure that it is detected and treated as early as possible. People who fall into high-risk groups should have their eyes examined regularly. It is essential that people with glaucoma have their condition monitored at regular intervals.

Glaucoma cannot be cured and vision loss cannot be recovered.

A variety of treatments can be used to help prevent future damage, depending on the severity of the condition. Most people with open-angle glaucoma are treated with medications to reduce the intraocular pressure.

In some people, medication may not be effective in controlling glaucoma, and surgical treatments (laser or incisional) have to be considered.

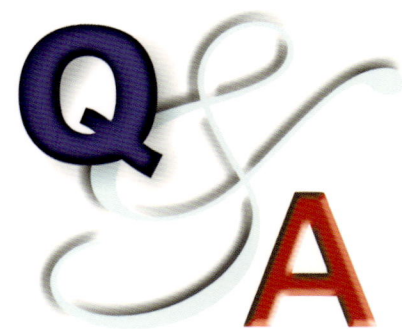

What is a cataract?

A **cataract** is a clouding, or increase in opacity of the lens in the eye, causing blurred vision. Eventually there can be a complete loss of sight, even though the eye's photoreceptors may be fine. Cataracts exhibit a chemical change in the lens rather than a growth on or within the eye. Some cataracts are congenital, but most are age-related.

Eye
(Anterior view)

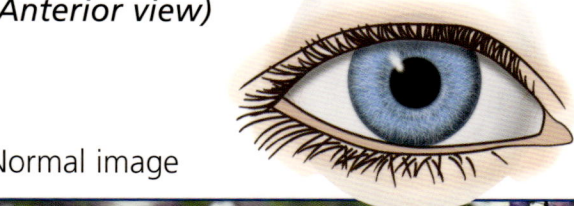

Normal image

Eye
(Anterior view)

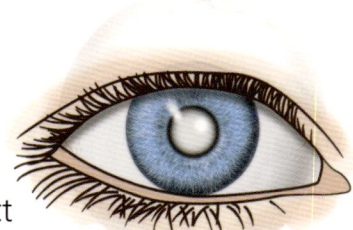

Image as seen through a cataract

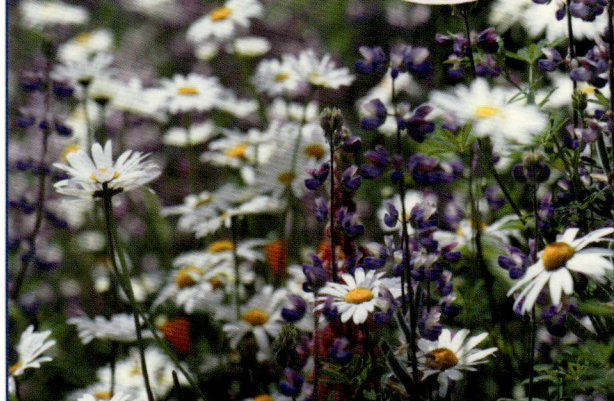

What are the symptoms of cataracts?

Generally cataracts develop slowly over time. Symptoms include:
- Blurred, cloudy vision
- Loss of contrast
- Glare, including halos around lights
- Increased need for more light for activities such as reading
- Sensitivity to bright lights, including automobile headlights

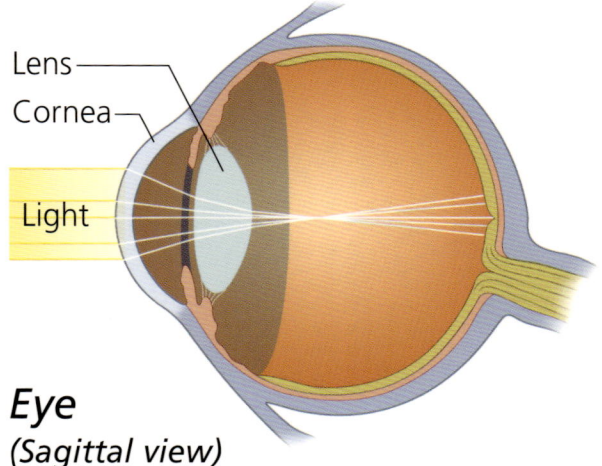

Eye
(Sagittal view)

Normal lens

One of the factors that influences the amount of **refraction**, or bending, of light is the curvature of the surface. The cornea is more curved than the lens, producing more refraction, but the curvature of the cornea is fixed. The curvature of the lens can be changed, allowing us to focus on nearby objects.

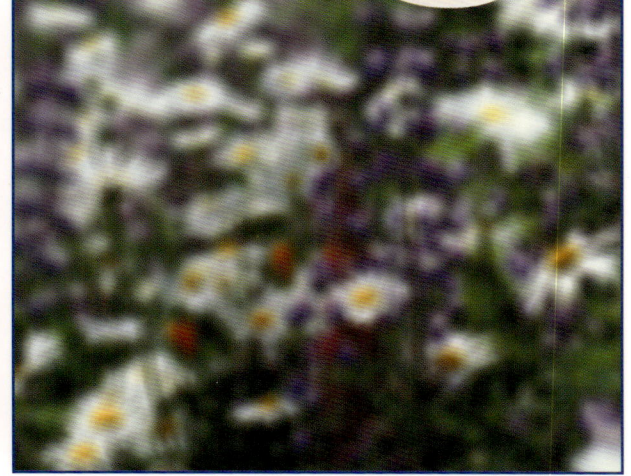

Eye
(Sagittal view)

Lens affected by cataracts

With cataracts, part or all of the lens becomes cloudy, causing the light to scatter, blurring the vision.

What are the risk factors of cataracts?

For many people the only risk factor is increasing age. Other factors include:
- Injury or trauma
- Smoking
- Diseases and disorders, like diabetes
- Certain medications
- Long-term ultraviolet (UV) light exposure, i.e., sunlight

Cataracts may begin in only one eye, but usually end up involving both eyes.

Q & A

Cataract types

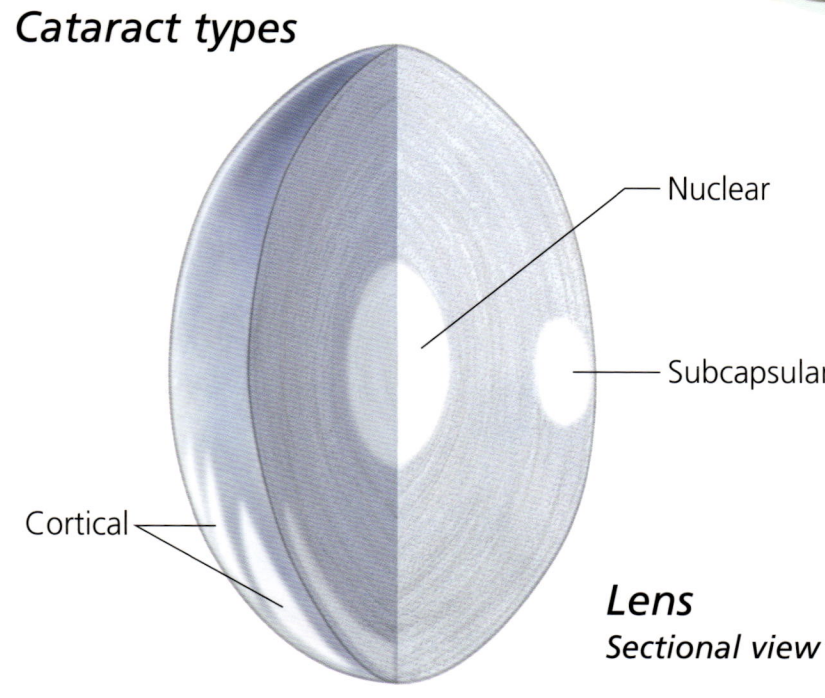

Lens
Sectional view

- Nuclear
- Subcapsular
- Cortical

What are the types of cataracts?

There are three major types of cataracts related to aging—nuclear, cortical, and posterior subcapsular.

Nuclear cataracts, the most common type, occur in the nucleus of the lens. With this kind of cataract there is an increase in light scattering, resulting in a worsening of distance vision. In the early stages near vision can temporarily improve.

Cortical cataracts begin as streaks around the lens' equator. Eventually the opacity spreads into the visual axis, impairing vision.

Posterior subcapsular cataracts are the least common. The opacity from these cataracts affects visual acuity more because they lie at the posterior edge of the lens, the crossing point of light rays as they exit the lens.

How are cataracts diagnosed and treated?

Cataracts may not be noticeable until they are advanced. The tests used for diagnosis are a visual acuity test and slit-lamp and retinal examinations. An eye doctor may dilate your pupil to look at the density of clouding in the lens.

Surgery is the only effective treatment for cataracts. Some indications for surgery are vision limitations during normal activities and vision improvement, if cataracts are the major reason for vision loss. Phacoemulsification is the most common cataract surgery. The cataract is removed, leaving the lens capsule and most of the lens intact to help support an implant. Another procedure, called extracapsular cataract extraction, may be needed if phacoemulsification won't work. In this surgery the hard center of the lens is removed, then the softer outer cortex is removed in pieces. A surgery called intracapsular cataract extraction, where the entire lens and capsule are removed, is rarely used. After cataract removal an artificial lens is placed in position

Early detection depends on regular eye exams. Steps to slow or prevent cataract development include:

- Smoking cessation
- Protecting your eyes from harmful UV light
- Eating a balanced diet with plenty of vitamins A, C, and E
- Limiting alcohol intake
- Following your doctor's treatment plan for your medical condition

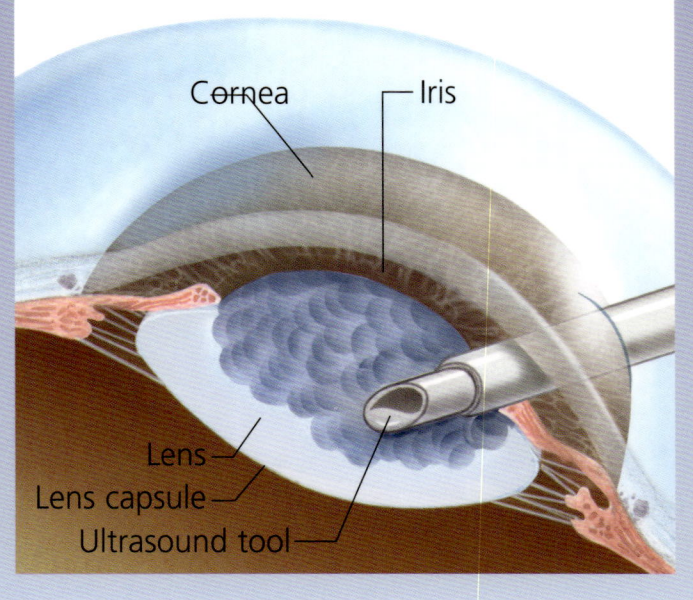

Cornea and lens
Sectioned view

Phacoemulsification
Removal of cataract

Using a microscope, the surgeon removes the cataract by breaking it up with ultrasound equipment. Phacoemulsification uses a very small incision and normally has a short healing time.

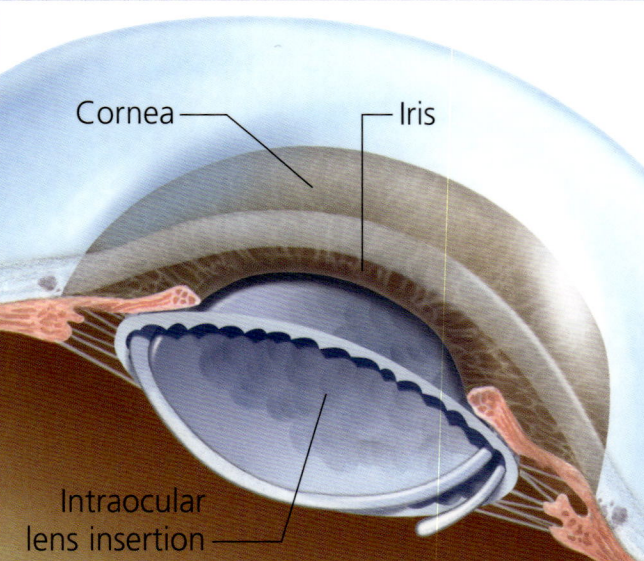

Phacoemulsification
Lens implant

An artificial, clear lens, called an intraocular lens, is set into the empty lens capsule. New lens can be folded, then inserted through the small incision.

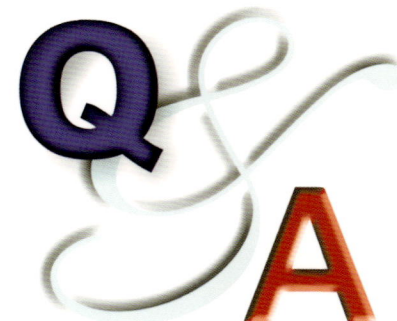

What is AMD?

AMD (Age-related Macular Degeneration) is a chronic eye disease that can cause irreversible loss of our central vision. Sharpness of vision comes from the **macula**, the central part of the posterior retina. AMD affects the photoreceptors in the macula, causing distortions and loss of vision in the center of the visual field. A leading cause of blindness in the elderly, AMD affects more than 30 million people worldwide and over two million in the United States. AMD is more common after the age of 50. Ten to eighteen percent of people between 65 and 75 years of age have some central vision loss from AMD. There are two types of AMD: dry and wet. Dry AMD develops gradually, usually with less severe vision loss. In wet AMD the progression of the disease is more rapid than in dry AMD. The effects are more severe, with the possibility of the complete loss of central vision. Peripheral vision is not affected.

Within the macula is a very small pit called the **fovea centralis**, created by a parting of neural layers. In this area incoming light falls directly on the highest density of photo-receptors (cones). The retina is composed of two layers: the thin pigmented layer and a much thicker neural layer. The **melanocytes** in the pigmented layer have several functions, including removal of damaged photoreceptor cell parts and debris, recycling a Vitamin A derivative used in the detection of light, and moving nutrients to the photoreceptor cells from the choroid vessels.

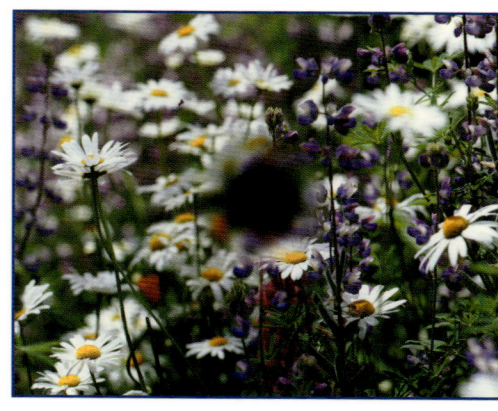

Loss of central vision due to damaged retina

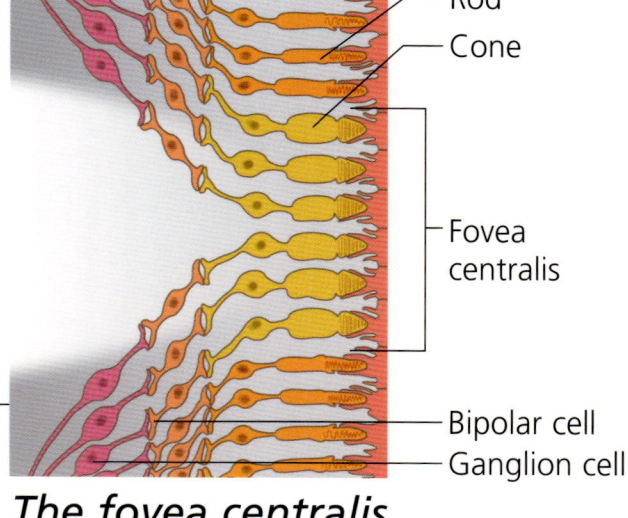

The fovea centralis

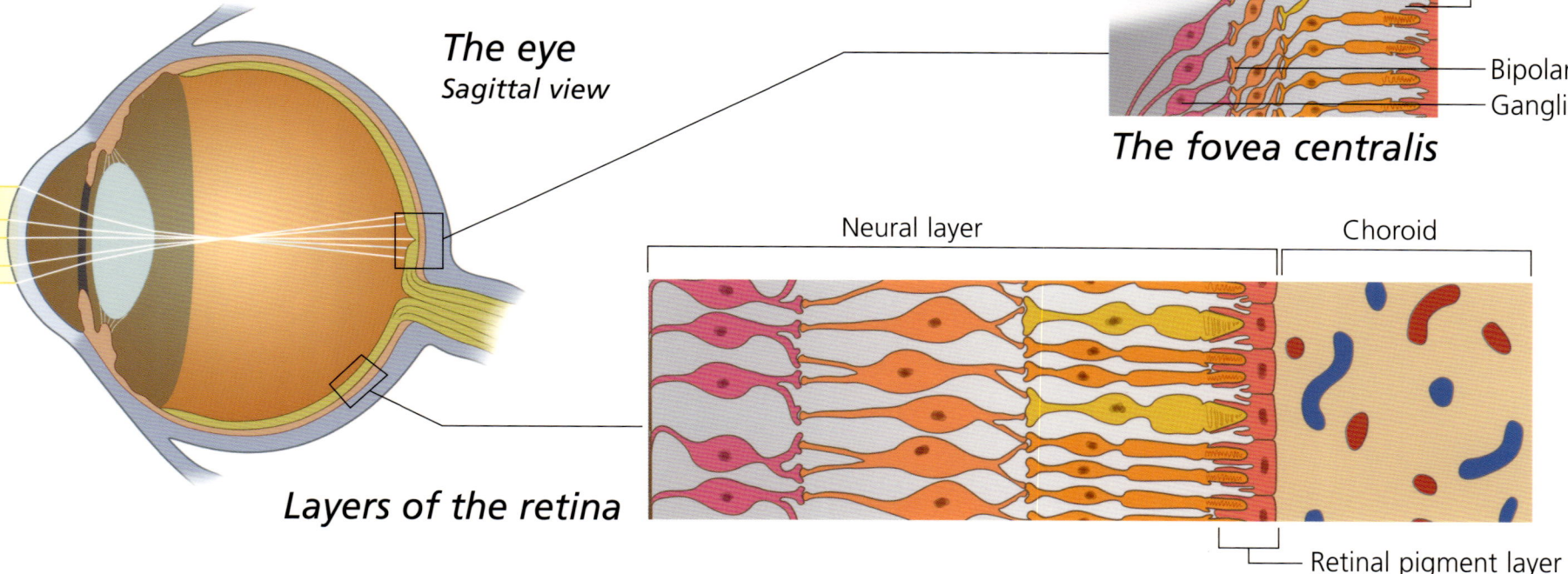

The eye
Sagittal view

Layers of the retina

What are the causes and risk factors of AMD?

The cause of AMD is unknown. Factors currently being studied include the role of inflammation and involvement of the complement system. Risk factors include age (the greatest factor), genetics, family history, smoking, and diet. Approximately 90 percent of patients with AMD have the dry version, with about 10 percent of AMD patients having the more severe wet type.

What are the symptoms of AMD?

Dry AMD (nonexudative):
- Gradual loss of central vision
- Distortions in the visual field, i.e., straight lines looking wavy or crooked
- Vision difficulties in reduced light situations, like doing detail work
- Difficulty reading
- Can lead to wet AMD

Wet AMD (exudative or neovascular):
- Shows all the signs of dry AMD
- Rapid loss of central vision, usually severe
- Sudden appearance of blind spots and visual distortions
- Blurred vision

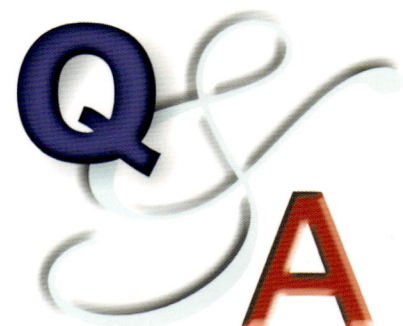

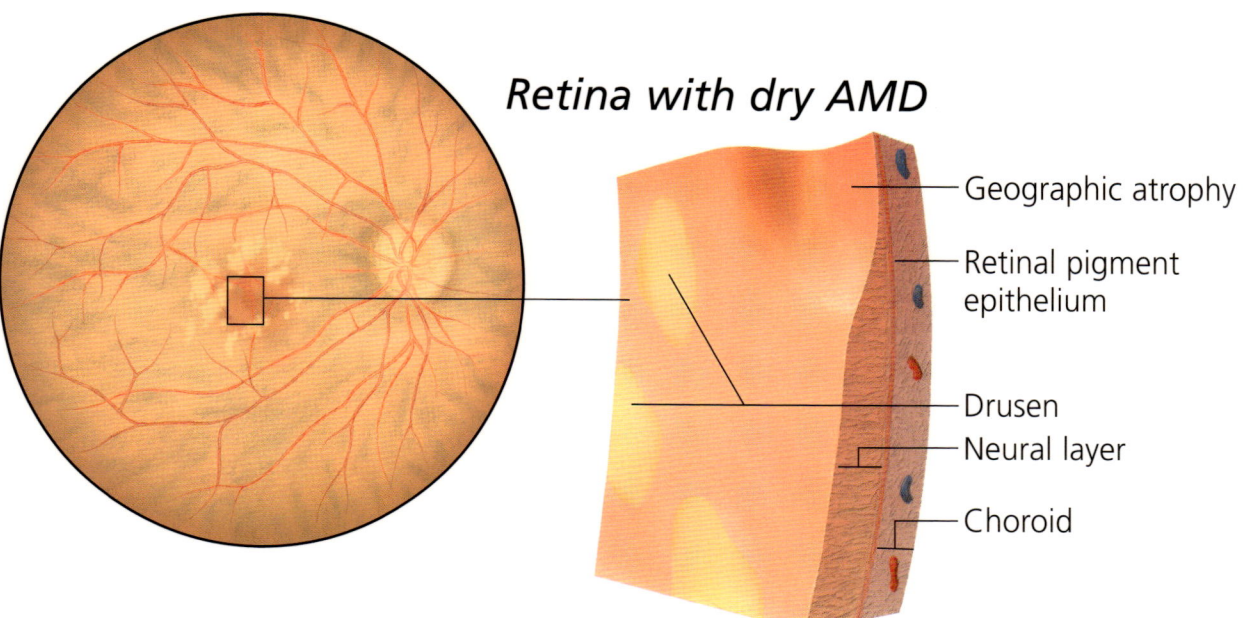

What is wet AMD?

Dry AMD, also known as nonexudative, involves the presence of yellow deposits, called **drusen**, in the macula. Changes in the retinal pigment epithelium (RPE) may be seen. Advanced dry AMD, also called geographic atrophy, shows depigmented areas, or the absence of RPE with visible choroidal vessels. There is photoreceptor loss due to atrophy of RPE.

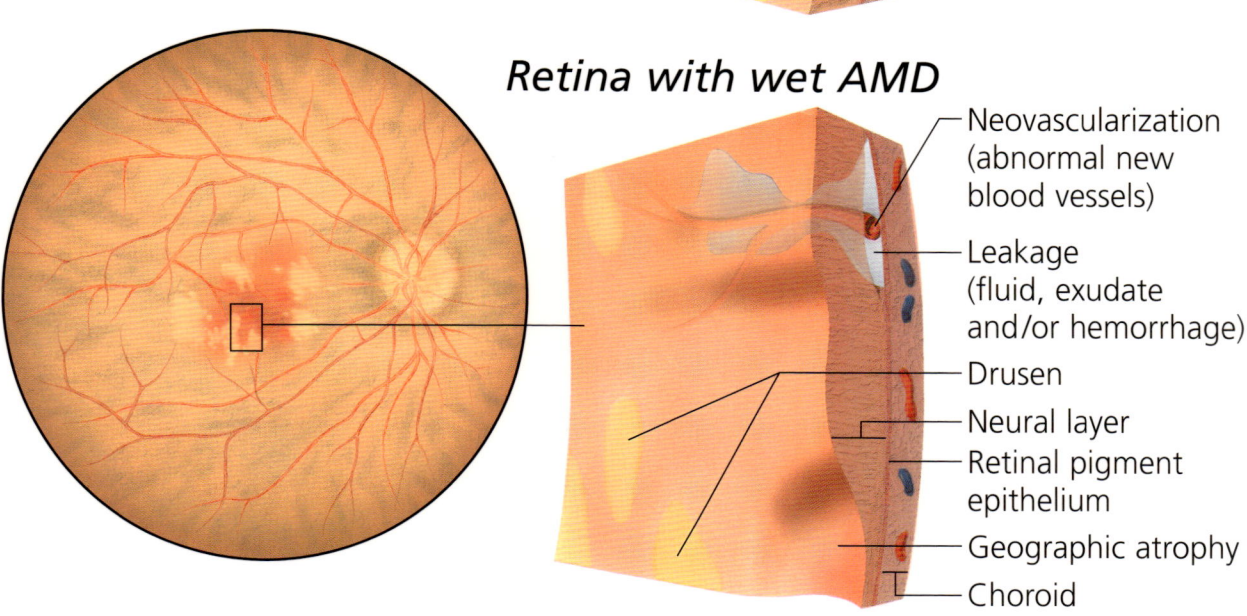

What is wet AMD?

Wet AMD, also known as exudative or neovascular, begins as dry AMD. Drusen are present, as is new blood vessel growth into the macula (under the retina) from the choroid. The vessels leak blood into the retina, raising an area of the macula, creating distortions (straight lines looking wavy). The leakage may cause a detachment of the retinal pigment epithelium.

How is AMD diagnosed?

AMD, is diagnosed through retinal examination using an ophthalmoscope. The use of an Amsler grid can help with the detection of visual changes. If there's evidence of wet AMD a test called fluorescein angiography can be performed. In this test a dye is injected into the arm. The dye flows through the bloodstream into the eye's blood vessels, and a photograph of the retina is taken. Another test, optical coherence tomography, creates a cross-sectional view of the eyeball, showing changes in retinal thickness and fluid accumulation.

Treatment options

Damage caused by dry AMD can't be reversed, but early detection and treatment may help reduce the loss of vision. One potential treatment for dry AMD focuses on slowing the progression of the disease through a daily supplement of specific vitamins and minerals. This treatment may also benefit patients with wet AMD. Intravitreal drug injections can reduce vision loss risk, and assist in restoration of reading vision in up to one third of wet AMD patients. Photocoagulation by laser, to seal off and destroy new blood vessels, may prevent severe loss of vision. Photodynamic therapy uses a cold laser and a special light-sensitizing dye to locate and seal off leakages.

The Amsler grid

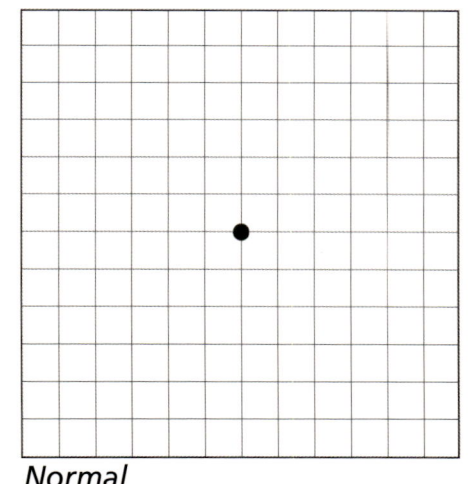

Normal

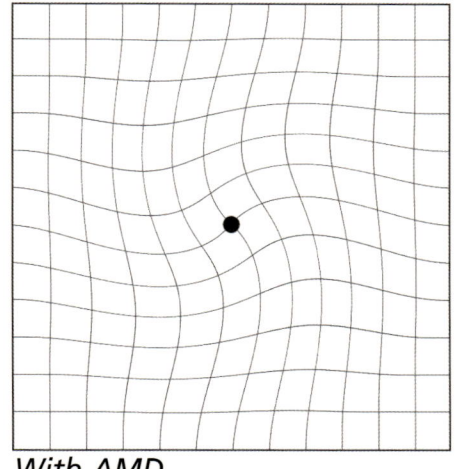

With AMD

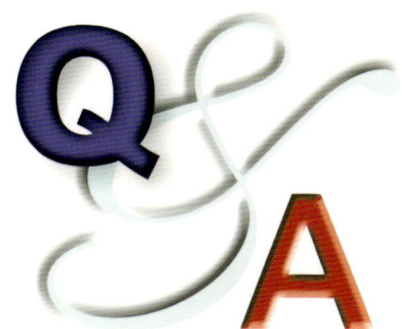

Practicing good eye health

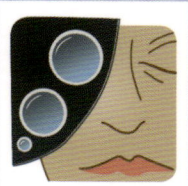
Get regular eye exams

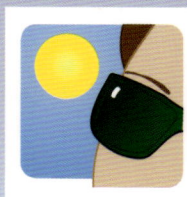
Wear UV-blocking sunglassses

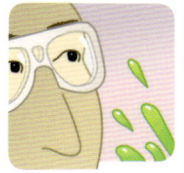
Wear safety goggles where appropriate

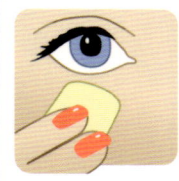
Be careful when applying cosmetics

Our eyes enable us to experience shapes, colors, and motion in our environment. The eyes contain about 70% of all the receptors in the body, demonstrating the importance of vision. Common eye injuries involve accidents while cleaning or working out in the yard.
Steps you can take to protect your eyes include:
- Getting an eye exam as regularly as appropriate
- Wearing safety glasses or goggles when appropriate, i.e., when working with tools or chemicals
- Being careful to avoid your eyes when using cosmetic products, including makeup and hairspray, be careful to avoid your eyes
- Reading and following the instructions that come with cleaning fluids and other household chemicals
- Taking care when working with car batteries, using jumper cables
- Taking care with potentially dangerous toys, such as BB guns.

During an eye exam a variety of tests may be performed. Visual acuity and visual field tests, refraction assessment, and glaucoma testing help evaluate your vision. In a retinal examination an ophthalmoscope is used to exam the **fundus**, the retinal surface of the eye. Changes in the fundus can provide clues, helping a doctor diagnose a variety of disorders and diseases, including glaucoma, diabetes, and hypertension.

How can UV negatively impact the health of your eyes?

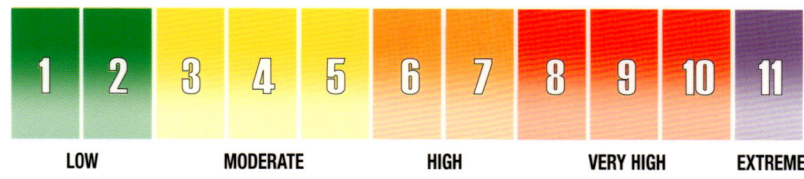

UV index scale
The UV index scale shows a forecast of the expected risk of UV radiation overexposure (from sunlight). The forecast is prepared by the National Weather Service, then published by the EPA.

UV radiation can damage your eyes just like it can damage your skin. Most people know that they need sun protection for their skin; however, few people know that they also need sun protection for their eyes. Everyone is at risk for eye damage from UV radiation.

UV damage to your eyes is cumulative and may be irreversible. Your eyes are exposed to UV radiation 365 days a year, even on cloudy days. Long-term exposure to UV radiation can damage the eye's surface as well as its internal structures. UV can increase the risks of certain eye conditions and diseases, such as UV-related cataracts, macular degeneration, growths on the eye, and even certain skin cancers on the eyelids or around the eye area.

Additional eye problems and disorders

Other eye problems include:
- Floaters – spots, hairs, or specks that float across the visual field; the most common cause involves very small particles suspended in the vitreous humor
- Detached retina – separation of the neural layer from the retinal pigmented layer; causes could be hemorrhage, tumor, or trauma
- Conjunctivitis – inflammation of the membrane that lines the eyeball; also known as pink eye
- Diabetic retinopathy – a major cause of blindness; the degree of retinopathy is connected to blood glucose levels, blood pressure, and the duration of the disease
- Eyelid problems:
    Sties – a painful swelling of the eyelid caused by an infection of an eyelash follicle
    Chalazion – relatively painless swelling caused by blockage of a meibomian gland
    Blepharitis – crusted, sticky eyelids caused by a bacterial infection of the eyelid edges